A Child's Suffering,
A Mother's Love

A Child's Suffering, A Mother's Love

Kimberly Cross Humphrey

To order additional copies of this book, contact:
Xlibris Corporation
1-888-795-4274
www.Xlibris.com
Orders@Xlibris.com
59761

This book is dedicated to first my son Trevor, for being my inspiration for this book, and also my husband Jay for his undying love and support. My Mother and mother in law, Margaret Jordan and Lee Ann Cross, for being my biggest fans, and to all my other children for giving me some of the funny stories to come in other books, Thank you Duncan, Colin and Hunter, you guys are great. Thank you guys so much for helping me achieve my dream. I love you all

CONTENTS

Chapter 1

A Mother's Story

I was a very loved little girl. I was taught the importance of family and what a bond like that meant. My parents were very supportive of me and my ventures, even when I lost interest and wouldn't stick to one thing. As I grew I was somewhat of a "pistol" some would say. I was a very rebellious child. I, however, wasn't lucky enough to not get caught. For this I am very thankful. My parents straightened me out, without even knowing it. As a teenager I wasn't very nice to my parents. As a matter of fact, I was pretty mean to my father, who loved me anyway. At the time I didn't understand how my parents could love me in spite of the way I acted and treated them.

I got myself into a lot of trouble, and of course my parents were there to try and bail me out of my trouble. But there were some things I had to deal with on my own. One of these things was getting pregnant. At eighteen I was pregnant and unmarried. My parents did the best they could to be supportive and I got married to my first husband on the twelfth of March in 1988. My first son was born, July 1, 1988. He was born with a neural tube defect. By the time he was six hours old, he was going through his first surgery. He had his first brain surgery when he was two weeks old.

When I was 21, and separated, I found myself pregnant again. I didn't know what to do. I didn't understand then that the love of a mother grows. But I made it and I gave them all the love I could. God made sure that the love I felt in my heart did nothing but grow. My parents helped out a lot, too. They loved my boys as much as I did. They did everything they could for my little men.

Eventually, I married again, to a very nice man. Together we had a pretty happy marriage, at first. A year after we were married, I was pregnant. He and I had two wonderful boys, Trevor and Hunter, only fourteen months apart. Both boys were born with an inherited disease known as neurofibromatosis. I will explain this disease later in the book. We ended up divorcing and going our separate ways. I don't regret it, nor do I miss the marriage.

I am now married to the most wonderful man. He has been a wonderful step-dad to all of my boys. I am very proud of my husband, Jay, and what he does to make sure that his family is cared for. Jay is currently serving in the United States Army. At the time that I am writing this story, he is on his second deployment to Iraq to support the war on terror.

As a Christian, I believe that God controls life and death. Trials and tribulation happen, because we live in a human world. Human beings are fallible. God never fails. His word is true and it will accomplish what it is sent out to do. All of my boys, as well as, myself and all my family, are in God's hands.

A parent's love is unconditional, I understand that now. My love will not die if or when one of my children passes. They will always be on my mind and in my heart. However, when our children suffer, our first instinct is to want to take it all away. We want to do anything we can to make sure our children are happy and healthy. When pain and illness racks a child's body, and there is nothing we can do to make it better, we have to put ourselves in a position to be strong for our babies.

I know that God is in control of every circumstance. I am not all knowing so I shouldn't presume to question God and his divine plan. All I do know is that God loves me and God loves my children. My love for my children will never go away, it has no limits, it is just always there. Yet, there are times when we have to trust God and not question his plan. We need to lay our troubles and burdens at the foot of the cross and leave them there.

Mothers, as a rule, tend to have a harder time with this when it comes to our children. We are constantly praying, "God take this burden, heal my child" yet we don't leave it there. We get up from the alter and pick up the worry again and again. We want to be in control, even though we want to trust God. What we need to do, as Christian mothers, is trust God to guide the doctors to help our children live. Leaving them in God's hands is the only way. Sometimes, God uses doctors to heal the sick, sometimes he divinely heals, and there are other times that God heals through death. This is a very difficult concept for mothers to accept. For some of us, our children are almost the only evidence that we even lived.

What we don't realize is that our children are not the only lives we touch. Have you ever smiled at a stranger? I have. Have you ever waved at someone walking down the street? Maybe just said "Hi" to a stranger. Maybe you have been there for someone to cry on your shoulder. Maybe you give to your church or a charity of some kind. There are many ways that we touch others. Just remember that you may be the only Jesus someone sees. We all, at times, get caught up in our lives and forget that there are others that cohabitate this land with us. We think only of our problems, and forget that there are others out there that have it much worse.

No one knows what I go through each day. As I said before, my husband is deployed, for a year. I have my eldest son, who needs some kind of surgery, another child about to go out on his own and make his way in the world. I care for my mother in law and I have my Trevor and Hunter that live so far away that I don't get to visit as often as I would like, and now Trevor is facing a surgery on his back.

There are people that I have met in my life that make me feel my life is inadequate. My life is difficult, more difficult than some people realize. Sometimes I get tired of being strong and I want to be weak for a while. Sometimes I don't want to hold all the burdens anymore. I get tired, broken hearted and frustrated and all the burdens get too heavy for me to hold. Sometimes I need someone to hold me for a while. Yet I still have to get my act together before I go to see my baby. I don't mean to say that any of my children are any more important than the other three, but he needs me to be strong not only for him but for his family and siblings as well.

Some people are really cold hearted that nothing touches them or effects their emotions. I want to know how to do that. Sometimes I think it is the only way I can be as strong as I need to be for my family. I want to have control of my emotions but the burden is too heavy at times. I really need help with them. In Matthew chapter 11 verses 28 through 30 Jesus said "Come unto me, all ye that labor and are heavy laden, and I will give you rest. Take my yoke upon you, and learn of me; for I am meek and lowly in heart: and ye shall find rest unto your souls. For my yoke is easy, and my burden is light." Sometimes God puts people in our path to help us. People to be his arms and hold us when we are hurting. The only volunteers I have to help me are my disabled mother in law and my eighteen year old son, who is about to leave. I am supposed to be their caregivers, yet they are there to be strong for me. I depend on them to help me carry the burdens that I have. I do have God to rely on, good thing he can handle it. In first Peter, chapter 5 verse 7 says "Cast all your anxiety on Him, because he cares for you."(NIV) I just have to learn to trust him, and not to pick it up again. That is much easier said than done.

As human beings, we want to lay it at the cross and let God handle it, but we want to have our hands in it as well. That kind of defeats the purpose. It ties God's hands and limits his abilities because we don't fully trust in him. In Isaiah, chapter 40 verse 31 the Bible says that "They that wait upon the Lord shall renew their strength; they shall mount up with wings as eagles; they shall run and not be weary; and they shall walk, and not faint." (KJV).

This means that we should fully trust God to do his job, so to speak. I know that God loves us and loves our children. So we should wait on His direction and His plan to reveal itself. No questions asked, no regrets, because, after all, it is God's plan. Even as parents we need to have the attitude of Job. In Job, chapter 13 verses 15 and 16, Job says "Though they slay me, yet will I trust in Him: but I will maintain mine own ways before him. He also shall be my salvation: for a hypocrite shall not come before Him." (KJV). Job is saying in this passage that even though someone threatens death, he will trust in the Lord. That he will always maintain his ways, the way he has always done things that gave him favor with the Lord in the first place. He speaks of God being his salvation, that people that lie and behave hypocritically can not come before the Lord. Further, in Job chapter 12 verse 10, Job says "In whose hand is the soul of every living thing, and the breath of all mankind." (KJV) He is answering his friends who have come to comfort him. He is telling them that God is in control of everything and that He, alone, gave breath to all of mankind. If God has given us breath, shouldn't we trust Him? I think we should. I am not saying that it will be easy to do, however, we should do it anyway. That is where faith comes in.

In Hebrews chapter 11 verse 1, the author gives the definition of faith. It says "Now, faith is the substance of things hoped for, the evidence of things not seen." (KJV). This means that in faith, even though we don't see evidence of what we pray for, we believe that it will happen. So, even though the circumstances seem to be continuing, we must have faith that God will work them out and answer our prayers. God answers all prayers. Sometimes the answer is yes, sometimes it is no, sometimes He says to wait. We should not turn our back on God because he doesn't answer the way we want. He, alone, knows what is best. I often use the analogy of a jigsaw puzzle. We know only the small piece of the puzzle that is our life, only God sees the big picture, because, after all, He drew it. Without faith it is impossible to please God, because anyone who comes to God must, first, believe He exists and that he rewards the ones who seek Him with all their hearts.

Noah, Abraham, Isaac and Jacob were all still living by faith when they died. They did not receive the things that were promised to them, however, they saw them and welcomed them from a distance. Faith is directed to the future and to God alone. Directing our faith toward the future and toward God keeps us from tying God's hands. Faith is believing that God is going to do what He says, in His time to accomplish His plan.

Having faith isn't easy, especially when you have an ill child, however, it is the way that God wants us to live. It is a lifestyle and something that you live. Prayer is very important. The Bible tells us, in Philippians chapter 4 verse 6, "Do not be anxious for anything, but in everything, by prayer and petition, with thanksgiving, present your requests to God. (vs.7) And the peace of God, which transcends all understanding, will guard your hearts and your minds in Christ Jesus." (NIV) God is telling us that, despite our circumstances we should not be anxious for an answer to our prayers. We should pray and give thanks to him for answering our requests and He will give us peace that we don't understand and it will guard us from severe pain. This doesn't mean that we will not morn our loved ones when they pass, but there will be a peace on us that will help us to deal with the situation.

Having peace with a situation does not mean that you don't care. There are times when I am faced with a situation and I don't know where the peace comes from, and I feel guilty for not hurting like others. But God promises peace that passes all understanding. I have felt that peace. I am feeling it now. I say often that I have a split personality, I have my human half and my Christian half, and a lot of the time they are at war with one another. The human half of me wants to break down and not go on anymore, however, the Christian half of me just keeps going, running the race and fighting the good fight.

I wasn't always as faithful to the Lord as I am now. I went through hardships and trials of my own. Some involving my children, some because of my own bad decisions. My life hasn't been easy, however, no matter what I did, God always had me in the palm of His hand. He always let me know in subtle ways. A gift from a stranger here, when I needed it. A kind word from someone there, just to let me know He cared. God has pulled me out of a world of sin and placed me into a wonderful life full of hope and love. If it hadn't been for the Lord, I would have no hope.

Chapter 2

Dealing with Pain and Suffering

Life is not about me anymore. It stopped being about me when I had children. Then my life was about my babies. When they hurt, I hurt. When something bad happens to them, I want to take it and make it all go away. But the Christian half of me knows that God is in control of the situation and whatever my children are is going through, God will use it for His glory and to accomplish His great plan. Sometimes we don't understand God's plan, or how things work together for the good of those who love the Lord, but God does what he has to do for his plan to work the way he needs it to work. God's way is not our way, but his way is always the best and perfect way.

I am a mother, I love my children with all of my heart and soul. Sometimes seeing my children suffer makes it difficult for me to cope with reality, but suffering is part of the human existence.

Jesus was crucified to bridge the gap between mankind and God, he suffered and died to save us. Why? Because he loves us and does so unconditionally. That means that it doesn't matter what we do, how bad we have been in the past, Jesus still loves us and died for us. In John chapter 3 verse 16, John says "For God so loved the world that he gave his one and only Son, that whoever believes in him shall not perish but have eternal life. (VS 17) For God did not send his Son into the world to condemn the world, but to save the world through him." (NIV). God needed to bridge the gap that sin caused between Him and mankind. So he sent Jesus, in human flesh, to be a living sacrifice and pay the price that is required for our sin. In Romans chapter 8 verse 1 and 2 it says "Therefore, there is now no condemnation for those who are in Christ Jesus, because through Christ Jesus the law of the Spirit of life set me free from the law of sin and death." (NIV). The reason that it was so important for God to give the gift of his Son, is because none of us are without sin. In Romans chapter 6 verse 12, the Bible says "The wages of sin is death, but the gift of God is eternal life in Christ Jesus our Lord." (NIV) Jesus didn't come to condemn us, but that through Him we might be saved from spending eternity in hell.

In Philippians 4 verses 8 and 9 it says "Finally, brothers, whatever is true, whatever is noble, whatever is right, whatever is pure, whatever is lovely, whatever is admirable: if anything is excellent or praiseworthy think about such things. Whatever you have learned or received or heard from me or seen in me put it into practice. And the God of peace will be with you." (NIV) In this verse God is telling us to keep our minds on good things, fill our mind with things that are praiseworthy and put into practice all that we learn from the Bible. I know this is a lot easier said than done, however, we must strive to be more Christ like. That is the only way that we can deal with the problems that come our way. This book is my outlet, to help me to deal with the problems that my child must face. He has gone through so much already, and doesn't deserve any more trials. However, God works all things together for the good of those who love Him. I have to hold onto this promise.

This book is going to contain a lot of information and inspiration, from all the family and friends close to Trevor and close to the situations that Trevor has had to go through in his life. I don't know where the Lord will lead me during the writing of this book, I just know what I want it to contain. I will give you the feelings of those closest to him and those that love him. There will be no negative feelings in this book. I will focus on all that is good, true, and right. The people in Trevor's life have not always gotten along, however, when push came to shove, we came together as an extended family and were there for Trevor. I must confess that, due to the fact that we are in the army and they sort of tell us what we can and can't do, I haven't been able to be there for Trevor as much as I wanted to be.

Being in the Army, we don't make as much money as people may think. So it isn't like I can just fly all over the country and do what I want. That makes it hard for me to be there for Trevor as much as I want. It also makes it hard to deal with the pain and suffering of being separated, not only from my children, but from my husband as well. So I will talk a little about how to deal with pain and suffering, from a Biblical perspective.

First, I will deal with the harsh realities of life. Sometimes we ask and ask for God to heal someone or us, and God seems not to answer or that He doesn't hear us. In 2 Corinthians 12 verses 1-10 Paul is speaking about hardships and pain. The reality of his situation is that Paul had a thorn in his flesh. He had pleaded with God on three different occasions to rid him of it only to be answered with "My grace is sufficient for you, for my power is made perfect in weakness." Paul goes on to say that he will brag about his weakness, or delight in his weakness and in insults, as well as any hardships. Paul says "For when I am weak, then am I strong." meaning that God uses our weaknesses to show His power. Sometimes we ask for God to take the pain away, but He can't always do that. Sometimes we need to go through the pain to prepare us for what God has planned for us. And God shows his strength when we are at our weakest. Jesus, who was God's only son, suffered and died, yet God showed his power through him by allowing the apostles he had chosen to see him for forty days. (Acts 1:3) God has called us to be witnesses to this world and show them the way to Christ. Through the Holy Spirit, God empowers every believer so that they can achieve this, even where they are at their weakest.

In Hebrews chapter 2 verses 9 and 10 it says "But we see Jesus, who was made a little lower than the angels, now crowned with glory and honor because he suffered death, so that by the grace of God he might taste death for everyone. In bringing many sons to glory, it was fitting that God, for whom and through whom everything exists, should make the author of their salvation perfect through suffering." Jesus was made perfect through his suffering and became the sacrifice by dying and being raised from the dead. Jesus knows the feeling of losing a loved one, remember Lazarus? That is the shortest verse in the Bible, it simply says "Jesus wept". So he knows what it means to suffer in the heart and in the body. Jesus was tempted, so he knows how we feel when we are tempted. So during Jesus' life he experienced every human emotion and every human peril, yet still died without spot or blemish. Take that in for a minute.

Jesus suffered, the apostles suffered and followers of Christ have suffered all through out time. What makes us think we are any different? Bad things happen to good people everyday. Just like good things happen to bad people. Romans 8:28 says "We know that all things work together for good to them that love God, to them who are the called according to His purpose." That does not mean that God picks on some people. It means that bad or good things God will work for the good of people that love him, who he called for a purpose. Believe it or not, God wants us all to come to him, so in essence he has a calling on each of our lives. It is up to us to choose to follow him.

Dealing with pain and suffering, from a Biblical perspective, requires that we first deal with the reality of what the circumstance is. That is what the story of Paul's thorn in his flesh is all about. Dealing with the fact that something isn't going "right" in our lives and striving forward. Once we do that, then we are faced with the question "When will it end?"

God's answer for this one is found in James chapter 1 verses 1 through 18. This talks about the fruit of suffering. That doesn't make much sense to a human mind, however, from God's perspective, suffering is testing our faith in the Lord. According to James we should consider it "pure joy" when facing trials. Although as human beings, sometimes it isn't that easy. My attitude changes in times of trouble. However, I always make it through the situation and I do always see it through to the end. Sometimes with the help of medication, sometimes not, however always with prayer and God always sees me through. Perseverance through trials is very important because it helps Christians mature and be complete, not lacking anything.

If we doubt that what we ask for will happen, then the Bible says we are double minded. To be double minded means that you don't fully trust in God's abilities. If we ask for something from the Lord, we have to believe without doubt, that God will do what He says He will do. Every human being is guilty of being double minded at some point in their lives. I know I have. The Bible says in Isaiah that by His stripes we are healed. I have claimed that promise and then turn around and let a circumstance overwhelm me. I then doubt that God is able to heal my child, which I claimed that promise on, and then when circumstances seem to get worse, I doubt His abilities. That is being double minded.

We are then faced with the problem of answering hard questions, or worse, asking them. How would you answer the question of "why" when bad things happen? In the passage of John chapter 9 verses 1-34 is the story of Jesus healing the blind man. A man who was born blind. When Jesus was asked who had sinned for the man to be born in this condition, Jesus answered "Neither this man nor his parents sinned, but this happened so that the work of God might be displayed in his life." Now this is a very profound statement. Jesus says that God allows some things to happen so that God can show his power and his abilities.

The religious leaders of that time, I think, viewed the blind man as a sinner and that his condition was a result of sin in his life, or his parents lives. Jesus' reply tells me that bad things just happen to good people, but that everything has its purpose. And sometimes the purpose is more important than the why. Jesus healed this man to show the power of God. He wanted to reveal who he was and at the same time, give the blind man a chance to exercise his faith. So Jesus healed him in a rather bazaar manner. Jesus spit on the ground and made mud. He then placed it on the blind mans eyes and told him to go and wash it off in a certain pool. After the man did what he was told, without question I might add, he returned home as a seeing man. The religious leaders of the time were very upset, because, to them, Jesus had violated the Sabbath.

So in order to answer these difficult questions, we must first ask ourselves: What is my spiritual sight? I have a few blind spots here and there, so my spiritual sight isn't any better or worse than my physical sight. Once we get ourselves in a position that we understand that God uses things for His glory, not for our convenience, then we can begin to seek, and find, God during our hard times.

In Romans 8:28-39 it tells us that we are more than conquerors. Our problem not being able to conquer something, some fear, problem, circumstance, is that we haven't exercised our faith. The Bible assures us that "neither death nor life, neither angels nor demons, neither the present nor the future, nor any powers, neither height nor depth, nor anything else in all creation, will be able to separate us from the love of God that is in Christ Jesus our Lord." That should give each of us comfort in times of trouble. Nothing in the world can separate us from the love of God. After all, that is why He sent His son in the first place. To bridge the gap between mankind and the Father of heaven.

Now what to do with all this knowledge? I will tell you, share it. Every chance you get, share the love of Christ with someone. Be bold! God allows us, our families or friends, to go through things in order that we have more compassion towards someone going through the same thing, or even a different circumstance, so that we can help them with their pain and suffering. During hard times when we are hurting, and we are in Christ, I find it very comforting that God sent the Holy Spirit. Why is that, you may ask. Well let me tell you.

There are many times that I don't know what to pray, how to pray, or what to pray for. It is in those times that the Holy Spirit intercedes for us. The Bible says in Romans 8:27 "And he who searches our hearts knows the mind of the Spirit, because the Spirit intercedes for the saints in accordance with God's will."

See? God set up a back up, so to speak, for when we don't know what we want to ask, or pray for. His back up plan is the Holy Spirit. The Spirit looks into your heart and mind and intercedes for you to the Father. Isn't that wonderful? I think it is.

So no matter what the circumstance, God has a plan and when we don't know what to do, He has a back up plan. Even with free will, that is pretty awesome. God has our backs, so what is there to fear? Nothing! As I write this book, I am writing it for everyone, but mostly for myself. I have to remember, during suffering or worry, that "For God hath not given us the spirit of fear, but of power, and of love, and of a sound mind." (2 Timothy 1:7 KJV) I have no need to fear for anything, God gives peace that passes all understanding, he gives us power, he gives us love and he gives us a sound mind. God is my rock and my shelter, I trust in Him.

Chapter 3

Cancer

Cancer is a term used for the abnormal growth of cells. That is very general. There are over 200 types of cancer, and then branches of those. When cancer cells begin to start growing, they "forget" to stop. The message that tells them that it is time to stop growing gets mixed up and they grow uncontrollably. People with neurofibromatosis are at more of a risk of developing cancers. Neurofibromatosis is an inherited disorder, characterized by developmental changes in the nerves, muscles, bones and skin. It sometimes causes lumps on different areas of the body, but is rarely fatal. Only about 25 percent of people with this disorder develop cancer of the brain, spinal cord, ear and eye. Neurofibromatosis also puts them at risk of developing pancreatic or kidney cancer. However, about half of the children and brothers and sisters of a person stricken with this disease will develop it.

Neurofibromatosis is also known for the lumps that present themselves on a persons body. These lumps are called neurofibromas, they are a non cancerous tumor that is comprised of nerve cells and nerve fibers in the brain. These neurofibromas most commonly occur in adults over the age of 40.

Cancers that occur in childhood are usually rare in adults. Cancer of the sympathetic nervous system is know as neuroblastoma. It is usually found in the adrenal glands, however, it can occur anywhere that there is a nerve ending known to be part of the sympathetic nervous system.

Testicular Cancer is rare and only occurs in less than two percent of the adult make population with cancer. Most commonly with males ages 20-34. The symptoms of this cancer can be detected early with self exams. The symptoms are lumps in the testicle, swelling, an alteration in consistency of the affected testicle. It may also include dull aching from the lower abdomen, groin or scrotum.

Primary brain tumors often start in the brain, as opposed to starting elsewhere and spreading to the brain. Brain tumors rarely spread outside the central nervous system, however, they can spread within the brain and spinal cord. Common signs and symptoms are headache, nausea and vomiting, and seizures. There are other symptoms depending on where the tumor is located which may include weakness or sensation changes in effected areas of the body.

Before treatment can even be discussed, a diagnosis has to be made. Cancer is diagnosed by several tests. A physical exam would be the first of these tests and should be extensive, including the whole body, as well as, questions about various body functions, and any changes since the last doctors visit. Another test often used is blood tests and tests of fluids and stools. Doctors also use imaging techniques including x-ray, CT, MRI and ultrasound, among others. Also a bone marrow analysis may be done. This is a procedure that involves a local anesthetic and a needle is inserted into the breastbone or pelvic bone. Then the doctor extracts a small amount of bone marrow, which is then examined microscopically.

Now, once a diagnosis is made treatment is discussed. Chemotherapy is the most common known treatment for cancer. Chemotherapy can achieve several results. One of these results is complete remission, where the tumor seems to disappear, which means that there was a complete response to the therapy. Although the ways to detect internal tumors are limited, they can miss tumors smaller than one half inch in size. So treatment should not be stopped too soon, because that increases the chance for relapse. Some remissions are temporary, where as there are others that are permanent. Remission can last for months or even years. Complete remission is not the same as a cure. A cure means that there is no sign of cancer for at least five years. Yet it is defined depending on the type of cancer and the patient.

There can also be a partial remission, which means the tumor may shrink by a half or more but not disappear entirely. While this is considered a good result, therapy should not be stopped until the tumor stops shrinking or disappears all together. If the tumor stops shrinking, there are alternatives. The Chemo program may be changed or surgery or radiation can be used to take out the rest of the tumor.

Next, there is stabilization. This is where the tumor does not shrink or grow. While this can be considered a favorable result, it tends to make doctors nervous, because they worry that the effect may not last long and the tumor will begin to grow again. The period of stabilization may last months or years.

Chemotherapy can also cause progression. This is where the tumor, in spite of therapy, keeps growing. Doctors are given the task of discovering this as soon as possible after the therapy has had a chance to work. Then they will begin to look at different treatments and work out a different plan.

Fear of treatment and of the side effects can cause problems with the treatment itself. Anxiety can actually make the reaction to the therapy worse. Patients also should remember that their body is not who they are. God determines who you are and that is in your spirit and personality. Patients then have the challenge of dealing with negative emotions. A lot of the time the negative emotions, when untreated, can make one lose their will to live and their will to fight. The negative emotions affiliated with cancer include, anger, fear, loss of self esteem and feelings of isolation. These should be resolved before treatment begins. Another source of concern for patients is the pain.

There are two types of pain, acute and chronic, and there are two sources of pain, physical causes and psychological components as well. Acute pain comes on sudden and is usually intense. Where as chronic pain, while it can be just as intense, the levels seem to rise and fall, but it never seems to go away. It seems to always be in the background. Always lingering. The emotional sources of pain can be worry and fear. Fear of death, fear of suffering, fear of deformity, or of being a financial burden on family or friends, or of being disabled or the fear of isolation. As you can see, there are many different ways a cancer patient suffers.

In Jeremiah chapter 15 verse 18 it says "Why is my pain perpetual, and my wounds incurable, which refuses to be healed? Will you surely be to me like an unreliable stream. As water that fail?" The lesson is that God spares no effort to bless us. He promised this. If we feel forgotten or too far away for God to hear us, God will retrieve us just to bless us. God, only, knows the human heart. We can not understand the deceptions and the dead ends of our own hearts. So when our own hearts condemn us, we turn to our maker. Sometimes the why is not as important as God's purpose for the situation.

Isaiah chapter 21 verses 3 and 4 says, "Therefore my loins are filled with pain. Pangs have taken hold of me like the pangs of a woman in labor. I was distressed when I heard it: I was dismayed when I saw it. My heart wavered, fearfulness frightened me." The lesson in this is that God wants to bless all people, He works world wide. If you remember 2 Timothy chapter 1 verse 7, it says "For God doesn't give us a spirit of fear, but of power and of love and of a sound mind." Which means we have nothing to fear. In Psalm chapter 25 verse 18 David says "Look on my affliction and my pain and forgive all my sins." the lesson in this is that God saves us for His sake and for His glory. It is not because we are worthy or that we are smart enough. God saves us by His grace and His love. We don't go to heaven because we were good enough, we will never be good enough. We have to except the gift of salvation from God, because it is the only way.

There are common and chronic side effects involved with Chemotherapy. The most common and immediate side effects are nausea and vomiting. These can be controlled with medication, but not without side effects of their own. Most anti-nausea medication causes sleepiness and general fatigue. Chronic side effects are a little more dangerous, or can cause a low self esteem.

The chronic side effects include hair loss, sore mouth and low blood counts. Hair loss can vary from just thinning to complete loss of hair to include all body hair. It may be sudden or gradual. The sore mouth is relatively common but only lasts a few days. Low blood counts have several effects depending on which blood counts are low. With low red cells, the patient would experience a general feeling of weakness. While with low white cells, makes the patient more prone to infection, this is commonly known as immune compromised. A low platelet count can cause easy bruising and bleeding. So patients with this problem should avoid getting hurt or cut. So to deal with the side effects is difficult enough. In order to properly deal with the side effects the patient has to take the right approach. They must, first, be informed that some of the most effective drugs against cancer provoke the most side effects.

So you can imagine how difficult it must be for anyone to go through any of this, much less a child. It just breaks your heart. Without God, these kids have no hope. But with God in their hearts and lives they can have hope. Hope for healing, or the hope of a new body in heaven. In Revelation chapter 21 verse 4 says "And God will wipe away every tear from their eyes: there shall be no more death nor sorrow, nor crying, there shall be no more pain for the former things have passed away." We should find comfort in these words for several reasons.

First, this life is not the end, and whatever suffering we endure here is only temporary. When we reach our eternal home, heaven, it will not grow old. Because God promises to make all things new. God loves new things. Our hearts will become new, we will always have new songs to sing. The best thing about heaven is going to be the presence of God himself. He will make all suffering and pain go away. So I can see how someone that is terminally ill would look forward to this day. The day they die to this earth. The good thing is that I have met several cancer patients, not just my child, but adults as well and even though they were in pain and felt really badly, they never complained and looked at each day as a blessing.

That is the way we should be. God made us to praise him and, actually, we are all on borrowed time. God gives us each day and we should make the most of it and rejoice and be glad for what we have. In Psalm 29:11 David writes "The Lord will give strength unto his people; the Lord will bless his people with peace." Then in chapter 30 of Psalm verses 11 and 12 he says "Thou hast turned for me my mourning into dancing: thou hast put off my sackcloth, and girded me with gladness. To the end that my glory may sing praise to thee, and not be silent. O Lord my God, I will give thanks unto thee for ever."

Chapter 4

Prayer, Why is it so Important?

Prayer is important for several different reasons. We have to learn how to pray, what is important to say, what God wants to hear from us and how we should ask for things. The first reason for prayer is communion with God through Christ. Simply put, God wants us to acknowledge Him and He wants us to talk to Him. When someone accepts Christ as their savior, it is not automatic to know how to pray. For years I found myself praying for the wrong things, then getting angry because it seemed God wasn't listening. In all that time, I did not understand that God was listening, I wasn't being truthful and I wasn't praying for what I needed to pray for. So I had to learn to pray correctly.

Prayer is also used for comfort. In John chapter 14 verses 15 and 16, Jesus says "If you love me, you will obey what I command. And I will ask the Father, and he will give you another comforter to be with you forever." The Holy Spirit is not just to be a counselor, he is the comforter. There are going to be times that you are so distraught you are not going to know what to pray, well I have comforting news for you. In Romans 8:26 the Bible says

"In the same way, the Spirit helps us in our weakness. We do not know what we ought to pray for, but the Spirit himself intercedes for us with groans that words cannot express." The good news is that when we don't know what to pray, the Spirit that lives in us does. He knows your heart and your mind, and he prays with the language of the angels. He is our intercessor.

Now in Matthew chapter 6 verses 5 through 15, Jesus does much teaching on prayer. He warns us not to pray so we can be heard, not in the open where everyone can see. We should go in private, because the Father that sees in secret will reward you openly. He warns against repetition. Repetitive prayers are not as sincere. God already knows what we want or need before we ask, so why pray? Because God wants us to talk to him. We should pray in earnest.

Now everyone who has ever been to church knows the Lord's prayer. In Matthew chapter 6: 9-13, Jesus gives an example prayer. The key word in that sentence is example. Jesus did not intend for us to repeat that prayer from memory and consider it having a relationship with God. From that example, I have gotten a few points that I think Jesus was trying to get across. First "Our Father which art in heaven, Hallowed be thy name." We are to acknowledge God for who he is and hold him in holy awe, be reverent. Then "Thy kingdom come. Thy will be done in earth, as it is in heaven." This first acknowledges that God's kingdom hasn't come yet. The rest of this verse says, to me, your will is my will. I want to do whatever is in your will. Next, "Give us this day our daily bread." We need to ask God to provide for us everyday. Then, "And forgive us our debts, as we forgive our debtors." Jesus is saying ask for forgiveness and at the same time ask for help forgiving others. Verse 13 then says "And lead us not into temptation, but deliver us from evil: For thine is the kingdom, and the power, and the glory, for ever, Amen." This is simply asking for guidance for what may come your way, asking for deliverance from any evil that might come into your life and we should end our prayers by thanking God for answering our prayer and giving him glory and honor. Praise Him for who he is.

All through out the gospels, the Bible talks about how Jesus went away to pray. To truly commune with God, you have to be still, quiet, and alone. God wants your undivided attention. In the book of John chapter 16 verse 26, Jesus gives us a promise. He says "At that day ye shall ask in my name: and I say not unto you, that I will pray the Father for you" Jesus is saying that if we have the faith, anything we ask for in His name, He will intercede, Himself, for us and ask it of the Father.

Ephesians chapter 6 verse 18 says "Praying always with prayer and supplication in the Spirit, and watching there unto with all perseverance and supplication for all saints." This verse means that we should pray always and without prayer the armor of God is worthless. We should not only pray for ourselves, but for each other. The verse says "for all saints". Spiritual battle is not just an individual problem, it is a problem for the entire body of Christ. In 1 Thessalonians chapter 5 verse 17 it simply says "Pray without ceasing", this means pray all the time. Never stop praying, silently or out loud. Believers don't always pray aloud, however we should always have an attitude of prayer.

James chapter 5 verse 13 says "Is any among you afflicted? Let him pray." verse 15 goes on to say "And the prayer of faith shall save the sick, and the Lord shall raise him up; and if he have committed sins, they shall be forgiven him. (vs. 16) Confess your faults one to another, and pray one for another, that ye may be healed. The effectual fervent prayer of a righteous man avails much" We must pray for one another and for ourselves. The Bible promises that the "effectual fervent prayer" of righteous will have power.

Even Jesus prayed, and he prayed a lot. He prayed alone. His apostles prayed fervently and after Jesus was crucified and rose again, then ascended into heaven, he gave to his apostles all power to work miracles in his name. In Acts chapter 3 is the story of Peter and John going into the temple to pray. There was a man who couldn't walk, he had been this way since birth. People carried him to the gate and left him there to beg for money. Then Peter says to him "Silver and gold have I none; but such as I have I give to you: In the name of Jesus Christ of Nazareth rise up and walk". Guess what, he did, and then he went into the temple to praise God for his miracle.

Prayer is a very powerful weapon we have against the devil. Prayer alone is not enough. We have to have faith to go with it. We have to believe that what we pray for we will receive, and not doubt it in our hearts. That is what makes prayer so important during times of trial and hardship. With prayer have the faith to move mountains and be a prayer warrior. Pray without stopping, always be in constant communion with God. Stay connected, then you can make it through anything.

Chapter 5

Trevor's Story

On September 15, 1993 a wonderful little boy was born. He was a very loved little boy. Loved by his family, his brothers, his grandparents. As he grew he was quite the little prankster. When he was about 2 years old he started hiding things, and he wouldn't talk so asking him where it was became pointless. Although he made us laugh many days when we wanted to cry.

When he was a little boy, he was such a joy to have around. Always sharing his things and hugging everyone. For the longest time he had the most wonderful disposition. He looked up to his brothers and he was always full of questions, when he would talk at all. He had his little fascination with hiding things. There are things we still can't find that he hid when he was little. It was so funny. Now as I am thinking back to those days, it still makes me laugh. He has always been able to help people to laugh and enjoy life.

Trevor loves video games, he likes school and his friends. He also loves his computer. He knows more about computers than his mother, that is for sure. Trevor's initial diagnosis was neurofibromatosis. It was inherited from his father. Since that time he has had tumors come up in several places.

He was diagnosed with a brain tumor when he was seven years old that was removed. We were so afraid we were going to lose him then, but God heard my prayers and he pulled through that one. Trevor is a very loved child, all of my children are very loved. My husband, Trevor's step father simply adores him. He protects him when he is with us. Of course my dogs simply adore him as well. Trevor loves my "snow dogs", as he calls them. Both Trevor and Hunter love the dogs, and the dogs love them. My eldest dog, Ludo, lets Trevor lay on him while he is watching television. Ludo will not get up until Trevor does, I think that Ludo is afraid he will hurt Trevor if he gets up before Trevor does.

Trevor likes to sleep with the dog, even when it makes him uncomfortable. There were many times that he shared the couch with Ludo and let Ludo sleep on the other end of the couch. Ludo was an abused animal when we got him and so he has trust issues with humans. Yet, Trevor won him over in a matter of minutes. Trevor was never scared of Ludo, even though he was over 90 pounds, and has big teeth.

Trevor is ever the inspiration, he is the inspiration of this book. He is the reason I am writing it. Trevor has done many things that has been inspirational. He tells everyone that they should never quit. He also says that quitting is for losers. I find that really funny, yet very insightful for such a young man.

There was a time, we were stationed in El Paso at Fort Bliss, and my husband and his friends wanted to go for a hike up the Franklin Mountains. He was so determined to do it himself, he said "no momma, I want to go the hard way, I can do it." I just had to let him try. His step dad said alright but if you need me to help just let me know. To be a further inspiration, he made it all the way up and all the way down. Then he had enough compassion and determination to come back up the mountain to help his terrified mother get down. I was so scared, yet this little boy kept saying to me "come on mom, you can do it." How is that for compassion and love.

After we were moved to Hawaii, when Trevor was about 13 or 14 he was diagnosed with testicular cancer. He was so brave, he had one of his testicles removed and underwent a round of chemotherapy. He continued to be a happy child. All he wanted was to be able to be with his friends and family, but he was immune compromised, so couldn't visit with many people. He had to go to school at home and was so excited to go back to school this year. Testicular cancer is very rare, as I said before, and usually occurs in men ages 20 to 34, yet he, at 14, battled it with high spirits and a good attitude.

Now he has a tumor on his back, which started about the size of a pea and now covers part of his back, his entire butt and part of his leg. He is awaiting surgery to remove part of the tumor as to relieve some of the pain. To talk to him on the phone you would think that he was never in pain. He never lets on that he hurts as much as everyone knows he does.

For a child to go through so much pain and never let on how bad it is, is amazing to me. I have read a few things about his diagnoses and discovered that the things he has gone through are a rarity. That in itself doesn't make me very optimistic. However, I have to trust that God will guide the doctors and that Trevor will make it to be a man.

Trevor has a wonderful family. We all come together to do what is best for him and his brothers and sisters. His father is a wonderful father, and he has a step mother that has done a good job with my boys. Her name is Jeannee Booth Clement. She has taken care of my boys for going on 12 years. The reason she has had to take on this responsibility is not relevant, the only thing that is relevant is the fact that she "bucked up" and did what she had to do. I feel very fortunate that she has been there for my boys all these years. I wish I could have been there more, however, I can't live in the past. She is a kind, responsible caregiver and that is all that matters. Trevor has a brother and two sisters, that are Jeannee's children. I am sure that Trevor's problems causes her some concern, not only for Trevor, but for her own children as well. This makes us kindred spirits. We have that in common. These children didn't ask to be born, we brought them here, so it is our job to care for them the best that we can. Some things are beyond our control, for that we must have faith in God and trust that He has His hand on everything.

Jeannee has been an inspiration to me as well. I hope that I have been some help to her. She deserves to be happy and she deserves the best for her life and her children. I hope and pray that someday she gets all she needs and deserves. I had intended to do interviews for this book, however, the distance that separates the people involved prevents that. So I am just writing what I know and what I feel. Trevor and Hunter are special children, with very special families. They are wonderful children, smart and very opinionated, which is fine. At least they will be fighting for something they believe in. I only ask that they stay creative and live what they believe. That they don't sell out, for anyone. If what Trevor wants differs from that of his parents, then we, as parents, should honor his decisions. He is fifteen now, and can make choices and decisions for himself. He is smart and as long as he stays informed of all of his options, the risks and side effects and makes an informed decision, I will honor that decision.

He is who he is, and no one should change that. God made him the way he is for a reason. It is that person that is going to fight whatever way he chooses to. I believe in prayer. Prayer is the most important activity in my life and I can not think of a better way to combat anything in this life than with prayer. God is still on the throne and he has everything under control. I believe that God will do what is best for my boys, and he will give me the strength to handle what ever is to come. Philippians

4:13 says it best, "I can do all things through Christ, which strengthens me."

Also, God gives us another scripture that helps during hard times, times of fear, to give us strength. In 2 Timothy 1:7 says, "For God hath not given us the spirit of fear; but of power, and of love, and of a sound mind."

When you find yourself fearful, or overwhelmed, say these verses to yourself. They do help. I have used them for years, however, I am human and find myself still becoming fearful. I just have to keep reminding myself that God is not the author of fear, Satan is, and that God will strengthen me when I need it the most. God always has my best interest in mind, as well as the best interest of His plan. So there is nothing that can come my way that God and I together can't handle. I would like to remind my son of this as well. Trevor, no matter what comes your way, it will never be too hard for God and you to handle. Trust in Him with all your heart, do not rely on your understanding, acknowledge Him always and He will direct your path.

Trevor is not that difficult. He has very specific goals and dreams. All he wants to do is be able to play with his brothers and sisters. He wants to be as normal as he can be, and not let all this affect him adversely. He wants to be his own man without all the distraction of cancer, tumors or chemotherapy. My prayer is that, one day he will realize those goals and dreams. That he keeps his head up and his eye on what he wants, and does everything in his power to achieve those goals and dreams.

I also want him, and everyone else that reads these words, to remember to not lose heart, don't let anyone take your creativity. That is the way God created you and that is exactly what God wants you to do.

I just have to keep thinking and believing that God will somehow work a miracle in Trevor's life. I have to keep the faith, despite what the circumstances are telling me. That is not easy to do, I am human after all. The Bible even says that "Watch and pray, that you not enter into temptation: the spirit indeed is willing, but the flesh is weak." (Matthew 26:41). I have to keep watch and keep praying, even when I am tempted to let the circumstances take over how I feel and let them get me down.

Everyone that reads this book, take comfort that God is in control. He controls everything. Everything will work together for good. God's divine plan is in the works. We don't need to understand right now. When we are called home we will know as we are known. Right now we see dimly, but then we will see clearly.

My prayer today is that this book inspires others to keep the faith, even when things look bad. Keep running your race, keep fighting the good fight. However, don't forget to put your armor on. All Satan needs is a small opening to get one of his arrows into you. Stay in the word and in constant prayer. Remember the words God says in his word and know that sometimes we just have to be still. God already has it, and he will work everything out. We may not understand how he does it, but we don't need to. He is the one in control. He has done everything he can do to bring us to him, however, we have free will to decide whether or not to listen to him. As for me and my house, we will serve the Lord. He is my comfort, my shelter, my rock and my fortress, in Him do I trust.

www.ingramcontent.com/pod-product-compliance
Lightning Source LLC
Chambersburg PA
CBHW061222280526
45784CB00006B/2596